Complementary therapies: is there an evidence base?

Fiona Mantle

BSc, RN, RHV, CertEd, RNT

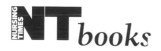**books**

Emap Healthcare Ltd
Greater London House
Hampstead Road
London NW1 7EJ

Nursing Times Clinical Monographs are authoritative, concise, single subject publications designed to provide a critical review of material that will be of value to practising nurses, midwives and health visitors. Their authors, all experts in their field, are asked to be challenging and thought-provoking and to stimulate reflection on current practice. *Nursing Times* Clinical Monographs do not seek to be exhaustive reviews but up-to-date overviews; their critical and evaluative nature is designed to promote best practice through consideration of current evidence.

Topics for publication are decided by the editorial advisory board, with input from practitioners. Monographs are then commissioned as near as possible to the publication date to ensure that the information they contain is the latest available. All manuscripts are reviewed by a board member and a clinician working in the field covered.

At regular intervals, 12–15 new monographs will be published. They will cover subjects suggested by practitioners (see below) and any major new developments in the field of nursing care. Each publication will be on sale for a limited time, after which it will be withdrawn and, if necessary, replaced with an updated version.

Note on referencing: NT Clinical Monographs should be treated as books

Suggestions for future titles are welcome and should be sent to Simon Seljeflot at NT Books, Emap Healthcare, Greater London House, London NW1 7EJ

Study Hours

All *NT* Clinical Monographs have been given a Study Hours rating. This is an approximate guide to the amount of time it might take a nurse, midwife or health visitor with no specialist education on the subject to read and reflect on the article and consider the suggested key reading list. By doing this you can accrue Study Hours to help towards your PREP study days requirement. Make a note of any related study you undertake and keep a record in your personal professional profile. For your free Study Hours pack, call 01483 455040.

The Study Hours logo is a registered trade mark of Emap Healthcare Ltd.

Complementary therapies: is there an evidence base?

Fiona Mantle, BSc, RN, RHV, CertEd, RNT

The aim of this monograph is to provide nurses, midwives and health visitors with information that will enable them to evaluate critically the available evidence on the efficacy and safety of complementary therapies in order for them to give their patients and clients informed advice and enable them to make informed choices about complementary health care. The review is not exhaustive and is confined to the therapies most commonly used by nurses in health care settings. The monograph is not about undertaking research into complementary therapies, nor does it cover the implementation of the therapies or nurses' professional and legal responsibilities since these have been well covered elsewhere (Darley, 1995; Rankin-Box, 1995; Trevelyan and Booth, 1994; Mantle, 1997; Knape, 1998)

Why do we need evidence-based care?

Twenty-five years ago, Cochrane published his report on *Efficiency and Effectiveness,* which stimulated discussion and examination of the clinical effectiveness of medical interventions. A key finding of the report was that the supposed value of some of the most commonly used procedures and therapies was not confirmed by research findings (Grayson, 1997).

Eddy and Billings, cited in Buckman and Sabbagh (1993) determined that around only 15% of medical practice was based on scientific research. From these foundations the movement towards evidence-based practice was established.

The medical maxim 'First, do no harm' and the UKCC *Code of Professional Conduct* both make it clear that the care given to patients by nurses must have a sound rationale for its use. This is enshrined in legal precepts in that, under common law, nurses have a duty of care to patients to promote safety and efficacy. In addition, the UKCC has discussed the use of complementary therapies in its guidelines on the administration of medicines and determined that the use of complementary therapies should be based on available knowledge and skill (UKCC, 1992).

What is evidence-based practice?

Sackett et al (1996) defined evidence-based practice as 'the conscientious, explicit and judicious use of current best evidence in making decisions about individual patients . . . by integrating individual clinical experience with the best available clinical evidence'. It is encouraging to note that the authors considered that the proficiency and judgement acquired through clinical experience were useful and valid sources of evidence. However, they went on to state that neither clinical experience nor the best external evidence was good enough on its own and pointed out that without clinical expertise, however excellent the external evidence might be, it might be inapplicable or inappropriate for an individual patient.

This was echoed by Castledine (1997) who emphasised the 'integration of the best knowledge with the practitioner's best clinical judgement'. He further pointed out that where there was little research-based evidence it was up to nurses to use their judgement based on what information was available. Among the evidence to be considered, Castledine included information gained from a patient stating that 'there is no substitute for a nurse's clinical judgment based on what the patient has to say, for this is often the best evidence of all'.

Evidence-based practice is a key component in clinical effectiveness. which the NHS Executive defines as 'the extent to which specific clinical interventions . . . do what they are intended to do, that is, to maintain and improve health and achieve the greatest possible health gain from available resources' (NHS Executive, 1996a). The RCN has defined evidence-based practice as 'doing the right thing in the right way and at the right time for the right patient' (1996).

So is there evidence to suggest that complementary therapies can be regarded as clinically effective? Contrary to popular opinion, there is a wealth of research covering a wide range of therapies. Muir Gray (1997) listed the following criteria for evaluating a therapeutic intervention:

- Effectiveness;
- Safety;
- Patient acceptability and satisfaction;
- Cost-effectiveness;
- Appropriateness.

From the definition offered by Sackett et al (1996) it can be seen that evidence of efficacy may be gleaned from a number of sources, such as tradition, empirical evidence, research, reported observation and survey which gives validity to clinical experience.

Muir Gray (1997) stated that 'many health care decisions must be made for which there is no high quality evidence . . . which does not make evidence-based decision-making impossible — it simply requires the best evidence available' and went on to list five categories of evidential strength:

- Strong evidence from at least one systematic review of multiple, well-designed, randomised controlled trials;
- Strong evidence from at least one properly designed, randomised controlled trial of appropriate size;
- Evidence from well-designed trials, without randomisation, single group pre- and post-test, cohort, time series or matched case-control studies;
- Evidence from well-designed, non-experimental studies from more than one centre or research group;
- Opinions of respected authorities, based on clinical evidence, descriptive studies or reports of expert committees.

It has often been suggested that it is difficult to design a double-blind, randomised, controlled trial for complementary therapies because of the uniqueness of the interventions and the difficulty of designing a convincing placebo for therapies such as acupuncture, hypnosis, reflexology or Therapeutic Touch (Anthony, 1987).

Resch and Ernst (1997) argued that, given the right outcome measures, even the most holistic approach could be evaluated through the use of randomised controlled trials, but Heron (1986) criticised the value of randomised controlled trials for conventional therapies.

Altman (1994) suggested that the use of quantitative research without a scientific basis was deeply unethical, since it involved volunteers and patients in clinical trials, while Lewith (1997) questioned the generalisability of randomised controlled trial results in general practice.

Lewith (1998) suggested that a better approach would be to compare the results of an intervention using a complementary therapy with conventional treatment rather than with a placebo. A well-designed single case study can provide clear efficacy of an intervention (Aldridge, 1988; Ernst, 1998). As Leibrich (1990) pointed out in her critical evaluation of research methodologies for complementary therapies, there is nothing inherently unscientific about anecdotal evidence when published by a world authority which can yield valuable scientific information without the use of a randomised controlled trial.

The world's first heart transplant was one example. Others include Bettelheim's observations, made during his interment in concentration camps on the reactions of people living under extreme fear and terror (Bettelheim, 1986). From the neurological sciences came the case of 'HM', who lost his short-term memory following bilateral removal of his hippocampus to control his epilepsy (Scoville and Milner, 1957), although Vickers (1995) raised questions about the strength of this type of data.

Leibrich (1990) also offered a well-argued rationale for a range of scientific research methods suitable for complementary therapies, pointing out that no one method of evaluation should be expected to assess the effectiveness of all treatments. She suggested that the assumption that only one method of research is acceptable could lead to scientific stagnation and pointed out that there was a need for more research looking at trends in individual patients rather than differences between groups of patients.

Vickers (1997) offered an eloquent discussion of the paradigm concept and emphasised the importance of matching research design with the research question rather than the paradigm.

McGourty (1993) discussed how to evaluate research undertaken in complementary therapies.

Research undertaken by Evans (1991) involved a survey among anthroposophical doctors to ascertain their use and clinical evaluation of 18 anthroposophical medications. The replies were analysed and the comparable efficacy of the medicines based on clinical observations determined, while the value of the more negatively reported medications were reassessed.

The researcher noted that 'the nature of the evidence may be regarded as having an intermediate level of objectivity between the experience of the clinician and the objectivity of the randomised controlled trial'.

Evans (1991) went on to suggest that the data had a high degree of detail and practice relevance and, since it was grounded in practice, had greater relevance than trials undertaken in a more artificial situation.

From Muir Gray's (1997) list it can be seen that many health care decisions have to be made for which there is no high quality evidence but which are based on what Swayne (1998) referred to as 'informed empiricism', founded on experience and clinical judgment.

Nurses and midwives are already familiar with this concept, since it is the format they use in their day-to-day work. Midwives assess a baby's apgar score at one minute after birth and, based on their own clinical experience, reassess it after five minutes. Nurses assess their patient's condition while using the nursing process, initiate a nursing or medical intervention and then re-assess and evaluate the outcome based on their experience, knowledge and clinical judgement or 'informed empiricism'.

However, since the information contained in many complementary therapy textbooks is based on the opinion of an 'expert' in the field this begs the question as to how far nurses are prepared to accept such information and, if difficulties arise, whether these 'experts' should be called to account in a court of law.

It is essential that practitioners should evaluate critically the research described in this monograph and decide for themselves the evidential strength with which they feel comfortable.

Unfortunately, one theme echoes throughout — comments related to the predominately poor methodological design of the existing research and, specifically, the small number of subjects or poor selection criteria.

Safety

Safety can be defined as meaning secure, protected, not involving risk — which raises the issue of whether any human activity can be truly defined as

NT *monographs*

Notes

being without risk. A potential risk can be assessed in two ways — relative risk and absolute risk. The risk associated with an intervention is the 'probability' that an adverse effect will occur. Probability is something that is likely to happen and implies a higher potential than 'possible'.

In these terms, a review of the literature suggests that, on the whole, complementary therapies sustain a high level of safety. Bach flower remedies and homoeopathy are thought to be completely safe (Spoerke, 1989), and hypnosis is safe when used by a properly trained therapist (Coe and Ryken, 1979).

Ernst and Barnes (1998) discussed methods for ensuring the safety of complementary therapies and listed the classification of adverse effects used in conventional medicine, which are classified into four different categories as follows:

- Type A — pharmacologically predictable; usually dose-dependent; can often be anticipated and prevented;
- Type B — idiosyncratic reactions, not predictable on the basis of pharmacological properties; not dose-dependent; usually rare; often serious and potentially fatal;
- Type C — develop during long-term therapy; usually predictable;
- Type D — delayed effects, such as carcinogenicity and teratogenicity.

Ernst and Barnes suggested that herbal remedies, aromatherapy and homoeopathic medicines could also be classified using the system. The authors felt, however, that the more physical therapies, such as acupuncture, manipulation and massage, were not so easily classified.

It can be deduced that if harm is done it can usually be attributed to the practitioner rather than the therapy itself. Ernst and Barnes also suggested that a further category of adverse effect would be pertinent in complementary medicine which would relate to practitioners' insufficient medical competence, although why this category should be confined to complementary therapists is not at all clear.

A review of the reported side-effects from acupuncture by Rampes and James (1995) listed a total of 395 incidents. However, these were collated worldwide over 20 years and included such minor reactions as syncope, bruising and pain. The largest categories were hepatitis (which can be eliminated by the use of disposable needles), drowsiness, syncope and pneumothorax.

Another report of adverse reactions from a Norwegian study again indicated that pneumothorax and fainting during treatment were the predominant adverse reactions to acupuncture.

Of particular concern for nurses is the confusion surrounding the therapeutic values, methods of dispensing and safety of aromatherapy oils and, in particular, what constitutes toxicity (Mantle, 1996; Vickers, 1996).

Fowler and Wall (1997; 1998) attempted to address this by relating aromatherapy to the Control of Substances Hazardous to Health (COSHH) and Chemical Hazard Information and Packaging (CHIPS) regulations. Unfortunately, even with this initiative confusions and conflicts arise. For example, Fowler and Wall referred to an alleged incident of hypersensitivity to citrus oils and pointed out that occupational dermatitis had been identified among workers who were regularly in contact with lemon and orange peel. This begs the question as to what the relationship is between workers being in contact with the substance all day and one drop of essential oil diluted in 10ml of carrier oil.

Fowler and Wall also pointed out that some essential oils contain phenols, which are harmful to health. Again the quantities involved in aromatherapy and the amount of neat phenol contained are minute in comparison with the amount of phenol in, say, red wine.

One of the key problems among therapies of all forms are problems that are not predictable on the basis of pharmacological properties, are not dose-dependent and usually rare, with serious and often fatal results.

The literature abounds with reports of this type of adverse reaction, from mild skin reactions to more florid manifestations. It would be a pity if therapies were to be banned because of these occurrences when many people are allergic to everyday substances — such as eggs, milk or feathers — none of which have been designated as dangerous to health or banned from public use.

One of the key problems in policing the effects of complementary therapies is the absence of an adverse reaction reporting system similar to the medical 'yellow card' system, which has been in place since 1964.

Although there are many complementary therapies practised today, this monograph concentrates on those which practitioners most commonly use in practice, those that could most easily be incorporated into care or those patients are most likely to inquire about.

Reflex zone therapy

Reflexology involves a range of techniques. Botting (1997) listed traditional reflexology (Ingham, 1984), holistic multidimensional reflexology, (Ashkenazi, 1993), reflex zone therapy (Goodwin, 1992) and vacu-reflexology (Griffiths, 1995) in her comprehensive paper.

She reviewed the available research on reflexology, starting with anecdotal evidence from a range of practitioners addressing the treatment of chronic conditions such as multiple sclerosis (Ashkenazi, 1993). Other long-standing conditions that responded well to reflexology included back pain, (Bosiger, 1989), menstrual disorders (Barron, 1990), asthma and anxiety (Goodwin, 1992).

Oleson and Flocco (1993) undertook a placebo-controlled clinical trial into the effect of reflexology on premenstrual tension. The placebo condition in this research involved the stimulation of non-relevant reflex points while the experimental group received relevant reflex-point stimulation on the foot.

Baseline observations were taken for two months before the start of the study and the participants were not aware to which experimental group they were assigned. Unfortunately there was a large drop-out rate (33 subjects from a total of 83), which left a small number of participants. However, results indicated that reflexology appeared to be effective in reducing premenstrual symptoms.

Lafuente et al (1990) investigated the effect of reflexology on headaches, using reflexology and 'medication', in the form of a glucose placebo, which was compared with prophylactic treatment with Flunarizin and a non-specific foot massage. The trial was conducted over a three-month period and, although there was no difference between the two groups in terms of headache prevention, it would seem that the reflexology was as good as Flunarizin as a prophylactic and had the advantage of involving fewer side-effects.

However, the study had a number of flaws, including lack of information about the age of the subjects, the type of headache experienced and the final small sample size.

Bosiger (1989) described the use of vacu-reflexology in the treatment of back pain. The treatment was effective on all types of back pain, complete relief being obtained following one to 10 weekly treatments, although no long-term follow-up was reported. However, caution is needed in interpreting these results, since back pain may also resolve without any treatment.

Motha and McGrath (1994) used reflexology on 64 pregnant women although only 37 women completed all 10 treatments. Their results indicated that reflexology may result in a shorter labour as well as a reduction in other physical symptoms.

Hypnotherapy

Hypnosis, which can best be described as the therapeutic use of the daydreaming state, has long been researched by clinical psychologists. The British Society for Experimental and Clinical Hypnosis has a useful data bank of research.

Since it is difficult to find a therapeutic approach that would constitute a placebo effect in hypnosis, most clinical trials compare hypnosis with another form of treatment. For example, there are several single-case reports (Olness and Gardner, 1978; Tilton, 1980) on the treatment of enuresis, as well as a number of comparison trials comparing hypnosis with conventional treatments.

Olness (1975) taught self-hypnosis for the treatment of enuresis to 40 children aged four to 16. Results after one month showed that 31 of the children had stopped bed-wetting and six others had improved. Failure to gain bladder control was identified as being due to lack of practice and the presence of a secondary gain, such as being allowed to sleep in a parent's bed after bed-wetting.

Kohen et al (1984) reviewed data on the treatment of 257 children with enuresis who were hypnotised after they had already tried other treatments for the condition without success. Out of this group, 44% achieved complete dryness, while another 31% experienced considerable improvement.

Hypnosis has also been used successfully in the treatment of childhood insomnia (Porter, 1975; Levine, 1980).

Clinical trials using hypnosis in the treatment of asthma have shown good results (Morrison, 1988; Ever-Stewart, 1986). The latter study showed a 26% reduction in the use of bronchodilators after patients underwent a six-week course of hypnotherapy. In Morrison's (1988) study, 16 people with chronic asthma were treated with hypnosis. After a year of therapy admissions to hospital had fallen from an average of 44 instances to 13.

Hypnosis is particularly good at addressing the underlying emotional aspects of asthma and helps in re-establishing the patient's control over the condition.

It is also helpful in the treatment of nicotine addiction, where lack of social confidence and peer pressure may be a factor. Lewith (1995) suggested that, as a treatment for nicotine addiction,

hypnosis was safe and as good as nicotine replacement therapy.

The range of conditions for which hypnosis has been seen to be helpful includes behavioural disorders, such as soiling, school phobias, fear of injections, pain and obstetric problems.

Aromatherapy

Aromatherapy with massage or inhalation is claimed to have an effect on a wide range of conditions, including skin complaints and infections. It is used as a muscle relaxant as well as a treatment for anxiety and depression.

Unfortunately a number of claims about the efficacy of aromatherapy are somewhat overstated and possibly even illegal.

There is considerable confusion about the lack of consensus among aromatherapists regarding the therapeutic properties, dispensation and toxicity of essential oils. This has been reviewed by Mantle (1996) and Vickers (1996).

Vickers noted that it was difficult to obtain any background evidence relating to the efficacy of aromatherapy and that a number of clinical trials were of very poor quality.

Lis-Balchin (1997) suggested that much of aromatherapy folklore was attributed to the fact that the effects of essential oils had been extrapolated, erroneously, from the works of Culpeper and other English herbalists and pointed out that the pharmaceutical action of herbs and essential oils was fundamentally different. She suggested that aromatherapy could help in some illnesses sometimes but that there was scant evidence that massaging with highly diluted oils would have any effect on internal organs (Lis-Balchin, 1997).

Buchbauer (1992) suggested that it was a waste of time applying essential oils by massage because of the evaporation time but that the preferred route should be by inhalation.

Vickers (1996) reviewed the research literature and particularly the two most commonly quoted works (Buckle, 1993; Hardy, 1991). Vickers

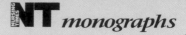

described Buckle's work as 'appalling', saying that it lacked inclusion and exclusion criteria, lack of baseline measurements and outcome criteria and of statistical significance.

In Hardy's work on the role of lavender oil in the promotion of sleep, the factor of rebound insomnia is not addressed and, while improved sleep may indeed be due to the use of lavender oil it could, alternatively, simply be due to patients returning to their normal sleep patterns.

Other research into the effects of lavender oil is more optimistic. Buchbauer et al (1991), using well-designed methodology, investigated the sedation effect of *lavendula augustifolia* on mice. Not only were they able to demonstrate a clear decrease in the motility of the mice after 30, 60 and 90 minutes but in further tests, following caffeine induction of hyperactivity, the lavender oil still had a significant effect in reducing the mice's motility.

Further research by the same authors (1993), again on mice, showed significant reduction in motility following inhalation of essential oils. Results indicated that the essential oils of lavender and neroli led to the most significant reduction in mice motility. In addition, lavender had the greatest effect on caffeine-induced hyperactivity.

Although lime blossom oil reduced motility, with the normal condition it amplified over-agitation in the caffeine condition and would, therefore, appear to have a stimulating effect. However, the traditional sedation effects of rose oil could not be confirmed in this study. It would seem, therefore, that lavender oil and neroli have a role to play in aiding sleep.

This effect was confirmed by Jager et al (1992), while Buchbauer et al (1992) further confirmed the sedative effects of lime blossom in normal and over-agitation-induced activity and passiflora oil in the over-agitation condition only.

Vickers (1996) commented that caution should be exercised in extrapolating from work on mice to humans, since human dosages are different.

This is an interesting comment since rodent experimentation is standard for orthodox medical research — a standard to which complementary therapists are exhorted to aspire. It would seem that complementary therapies are damned if they do and damned if they do not conform to biomedical standards.

Research by Betts (1996) is often quoted as an example of the use of aromatherapy in the amelioration of epileptic fits. The protocol involved patients choosing their own oils and using them prophylactically when they felt they were about to have a seizure. What is often overlooked in this study is the fact that Betts used hypnosis to induce an automatic conditioned relaxation response to the smell of the oil and the patient was then able to abort the fit.

One well-designed study was undertaken by Wilkinson (1995). It showed evidence that Roman camomile produced a greater reduction in anxiety symptoms than massage alone.

Claims for the antimicrobial activity of essential oils are better supported. Lis-Balchine et al (1996) described an *in vitro* investigation of the effects of essential oils against 25 bacterial species and three fungi as well as the pharmacological effects of oils on smooth muscle.

Their results supported the claim that geranium, neroli, patchouli, peppermint, lavender and marjoram had a spasmolytic (spasm-reducing) action on smooth muscle. High spasmogenic (spasm-inducing) activity was noted for bergamot, clary sage, lemon grass, fennel, frankincense, lemon and rosemary.

Antimicrobial activity was highest for tea tree oil, which proved to be active against 24 out of 25 species of bacteria tested and also had high anti-fungal activity. Other antimicrobial oils included bergamot, which was active against 23 out of 25 species, lavender (23/25), marjoram (23/25), melissa (22/25), neroli (22/25) and rosemary (21/25). The results from three varieties of thyme varied between 14—15/25, depending on the type.

This review of a selection of research articles on aromatherapy highlights the importance of good research design, showing that without this the value of a particular oil may not be apparent and its therapeutic value discounted, not because it does not work but because the methodology is at fault.

Massage

The role of touch as a therapeutic tool in nursing has been well documented. Beckwith (1993) suggested that the resurgence of touch in nursing practice was a response to the increasingly technical nature of the job and the dehumanising effect this can have on patients.

Massage is not a single therapy but a number of interventions that can range from gentle soothing movements to the deep massage techniques known as rolfing, which seeks to make structural alterations in the musculature and to liberate tensions.

Other massage systems might include stimulating shiatsu or reflexology points. Although some research designs are methodologically poor, Fulder (1997) pointed out that the main point of a massage is subjective experience.

Field et al (1992) researched the effects of massage on children and adolescents in psychiatric care and carried out a randomised controlled trial during which 72 subjects were assigned to a massage group or a group watching relaxing videos. Sleep behaviour, activity ratings and pulse rate were measured. Results indicated the value of massage: mood scores improved, anxiety scores fell along with salivary cortisol levels and, at the end of the trial, the massage group showed an overall improvement in sleep behaviour.

In Stevensen's (1994) study patients who had had cardiac surgery were assigned to one of four groups: one was massaged with essential oils, one with carrier oils, one had a chat with a nurse and one received no intervention. Results showed that physiological responses in the massage groups were transient but the psychological results for the massage groups were both clinically and statistically significant. Similar results were obtained by Fraser and Kerr (1993).

Thomas (1989) described how a simple foot massage reduced levels of anxiety in elderly patients and suggested that the use of a simple foot massage is a skill that psychiatric nurses would find beneficial to their patients.

It is not just adults who benefit from massage. Field et al (1986) gave pre-term babies weighing less than 1,500g 15-minute tactile/kinesthetic stimulation sessions that involved stroking and passive limb movements. Results showed a significant increase in weight gain for the treatment group.

Scarfidi et al (1993) investigated which pre-term infants would benefit most from this massage therapy and noted that babies who had experienced more complications before the study gained more benefit from the massage.

These two studies were carried out on babies who were medically stable. However, it has been noted that babies born before 34 weeks' gestation with respiratory problems do not tolerate massage well (Powell, 1974; Oehler, 1985; Harrison et al, 1990).

Although there are methodological flaws in many of the trials relating to massage — most of these are related to small sample sizes — they do indicate a trend that suggests the beneficial effects of massage in the reduction in anxiety.

Acupuncture

The main problem in trying to assess the therapeutic effect of acupuncture on a range of conditions is the fact that acupuncture is not one discrete therapy but a range of interlinked techniques that have been described as a 'multimodal system of healing with complex explanatory models' (Birch, 1998). It is a therapy which is constantly evolving in response to social and political pressures and, in doing so, has developed a wide range of diagnostic and explanatory models and interventions (Birch, 1998).

This makes generalisation from specific investigations difficult if the type of theoretical model used is not clarified. Consequently, the fact that 'acupuncture' in one instance does not 'work' does not mean that other models might not. As Birch (1998) pointed out, 'there is no scientific evidence to support the notion that one method of acupuncture is superior to any other'.

To reflect and validate the wide range of acupuncture models an equally wide range of research methodologies should be considered. Contrary to popular belief, not all acupuncture models adhere to a holistic approach and, again, research methods must reflect this principle.

One of the problems in acupuncture research surrounds the question of what constitutes an adequate placebo and what is the active treatment discussed by Birch (1997). He pointed out that what is used as a sham or placebo acupuncture can, in fact, constitute an active treatment, and active treatment may be quite inadequate to produce a therapeutic effect.

Other factors inherent in the evaluation of acupuncture research have been highlighted by Staebler et al (1994) who list, in addition to the placebo problem, the lack of control groups and the generally small sample sizes.

A review of the use of acupuncture for the treatment of chronic pain was undertaken by Ter Riet et al (1990a), who commented on the poor methodology used in the trials. In analysing the papers, the authors weighted the methodology of each trial out of 100. For example, randomisation was awarded 12 points, studies with groups of over 50 subjects 10 points — the larger the final total of points the better the study.

In spite of the poor research methodology, acupuncture was credited with having a role to play in the treatment of chronic pain. A detailed account of the effect of acupuncture on the central nervous system and pain perception was given by Benoussan (1991). Lewith (1984) noted that acupuncture on the whole was of value in the treatment of low back pain.

Lewith and Kenyon (1984) provided physiological and psychological explanations for the mechanism of acupuncture in the treatment of chronic pain, suggesting that it worked by modifying pain transmission at the spinal cord level and also by stimulating the release of endorphins in the cerebrospinal fluid and encephalins in the serum, both of which are naturally occurring opiates.

A review of the use of acupuncture in the treatment of asthma by Kleijnen et al (1991) showed equally inconsistent results with, again, an overall poor research design. The trials under scrutiny dated back to 1963. Since then there has been a steady build-up of knowledge which introduces an unwarranted bias if old research is employed to validate a therapy.

This has been commented on by Hammerschlag and Morris (1997) who, in their review of the use of acupuncture versus standard biomedical care, noted that there was an improvement in the quality of the research over time. They pointed out, however, that in spite of the low standard of research design, 20 of the 23 studies showed results that were at least as effective as standard medical care.

The authors noted specifically that in other studies acupuncture had a more rapid effect in relieving renal colic than an antispasmodic drug (Lee et al, 1992) and that it was as effective as the betablocker metoprolol for reducing frequency and duration of headaches (Hesse et al, 1994).

In a review of seven studies of acupuncture in the treatment of nicotine addiction, Vincent and Richardson (1987) noted that acupuncture was as successful as other treatments.

In a group of studies reviewed by Schwartz (1988) it was shown that sham acupuncture and real acupuncture were almost equally effective.

Ter Riet et al (1990b) also reviewed the use of acupuncture in the treatment of addictions (covering tobacco, heroin and alcohol), but suggested that the studies were again of low quality and concluded that acupuncture did not really work in aiding smoking cessation.

However, the rigour of Ter Riet et al's assessment was questioned by Rampes and Mortimer (1997). They challenged the validity of the scoring system when it was employed in their study of electro-acupuncture in alcohol craving. They also pointed out that Lewith and Vincent (1995) had commented that the discussion section of Ter Riet et al's review (1990b) of the effects of acupuncture on addiction was muddled and had challenged the credibility of Ter Riet et al to assess acupuncture as a clinical modality.

In addition, Lewith (1995) suggested that Ter Riet's main error was to confuse the question: did the acupuncture work or did it work as a sham acupuncture?

Silagy et al (1994) re-evaluated the research and noted that outcome measures were equal to nicotine replacement therapy, and the site of needle insertion was not important.

Lewith (1995) concluded that acupuncture could, in a non-specific way, trigger the release of endorphins that aid withdrawal in a number of cases of addiction. However, in none of these trials was there any indication that subjects' readiness to change their behaviour had been ascertained.

Therapeutic Touch (TT)

Evidence of the efficacy of TT is of very poor quality, although the value of empirical evidence must not be overlooked. Clinical trials have not done justice to this therapy, which is non-invasive, safe and easy to incorporate into nursing care.

Heidt's (1981) work on reducing anxiety using TT showed a clear reduction in anxiety scales as measured by a self-evaluation questionnaire in the patients given TT, compared with casual touch or a conversation.

This trial has been criticised for not having a placebo and for not being 'blinded'. However, it did fall into Lewith's (1998) category of comparable treatments, a well validated methodology.

Clinical trials in the use of TT in wound care were less convincing in the five trials described by Wirth (1995). The results were equivocal and key criticisms of the research design centred around subject selection and methodology. None of the subjects appear to have been assessed for nutritional status. Subject numbers in each study were small — less than 50 — and in one study only 15 subjects were used, covering an age span of 30 years (37–61), while in another study the age range was only 10 years. Subjects were randomised rather than matched, which would have been more appropriate in such small numbers.

Researchers often have little understanding of the critical mass needed for randomised trials. Randomisation with small numbers can easily introduce bias.

Krieger's early (1974) work is also open to criticism (Clark and Clark, 1984). In Krieger's study a sample of 64 hospitalised patients, chosen for the trial by their nurses, were given either TT or routine nursing care. Krieger's results indicated a statistical increase in haemoglobin in the TT group. However, what is not clear is the rationale by which the nurses chose the patients for the study, the ages of the patients, their medical condition and baseline haemoglobin levels.

Evidence for the exchange of energy theory in TT has been offered by Quinn (1982). In this study cardiovascular patients either experienced TT given by practitioners of TT, or mimic TT given by nurses who were unfamiliar with the therapy. The group who had TT showed a significantly greater reduction in anxiety status than those with mimic TT.

Unfortunately this has not been replicated (Quinn, 1989; Parkes, 1985). It has been suggested that since in Quinn's replication study the same nurses performed both the TT and the mimic condition and the intentionality of the TT was something that the nurses could not 'turn off' while doing the mimic TT, it was this which led to conflicting results.

Research by Meehan (1993) did not support the use of TT in the treatment of pain. Narcotic analgesia had a significantly better effect than TT. However, since the patients in the study had undergone major abdominal and pelvic surgery perhaps the hypothesis was a little bit ambitious.

Keller and Bzdek (1986) used TT on headaches with statistically significant results. A qualitative approach was used by Bulbrook (1984), who reviewed 15 case studies in the use of TT.

An interesting case study by Green (1996) gave a graphic account of how TT affected both her and her subject. A friend had classical migraine and, following neurological investigations and appropriate dietary adjustment, decided to try TT.

Treatment occurred once or twice a week. Green's friend found that her migraines lessened in frequency and intensity and that she felt more in control of them. This case study demonstrated the value of this therapy for both the therapist and the recipient.

It would have been even better if baseline measurements of frequency had been done and perhaps a quality measurement tool, such as personal construct theory, had been used. This notwithstanding, it is an excellent example of how empirical research into complementary therapies can be undertaken.

Cox and Hayes (1997, 1998) confirmed the effects of TT in the treatment of anxiety in a patient in intensive care.

Babies also appear to respond well to TT (Thayer, 1990). Fedoruk (1985) used TT to reduce the levels of stress in preterm neonates. TT has also been used to reduce stress levels in children aged from two months to two years. The group who had TT as opposed to casual touch showed a statistically significant reduction in stress (Kramer, 1990).

Summary

It can be seen from this review of the evidence for some complementary therapies that there are serious problems in the standard of the research. Common to many studies is the poor selection of subjects (often too few), the lack of clear baseline measurements and clearly defined expected outcomes.

These problems are common to many designs and not specific to randomised controlled trials. As well as having a poor understanding of research methodology, researchers occasionally display a lack of understanding of the principles underlying nursing or medical care.

For example, anyone who has undergone major abdominal surgery will sympathise with Meehan's (1993) subjects who found narcotic analgesia preferable to TT, while the healing effects of TT on tension headaches can easily be appreciated.

Lewith (1998) suggested that there were a variety of research methodologies, well validated in other disciplines, that would be suitable for researching complementary therapies and would enable researchers to break away from the stranglehold of the double-blind, randomised controlled trial, which tends to be time-consuming and expensive.

The sign of a mature profession is reflected in its ability to be flexible, open-minded and to cope with ambiguity. For the nursing profession to cling to the ethos of the randomised controlled trial just because the scientific community has designated it as some sort of 'gold standard' would indicate a profession that is still immature.

Nursing should decide for itself what its own 'gold standard' for research is, which means using whatever methods suits the research question rather than the method that is politically correct.

As far as complementary therapies are concerned, it would seem invidious to reject any of the therapies as a treatment modality based on poor research and inappropriate design, especially research carried out over 30 years ago when, for example, the mechanics of sham acupuncture were not fully understood.

However, poor research design does not do justice to the therapies that

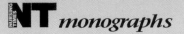

have stood the test of time, evolving and developing over the years; such research hampers the acceptance of complementary therapies, often unfairly.

Practitioners should continue to keep an open mind, since poor research design (using any methodology) gives a false idea of how effective an intervention might be. They should assess the evidential strength of the research as described by Muir Gray (1997) and decide for themselves the level of strength that they are happy with. **NT**

References

Aldridge, D. (1988) Single case study research designs. *Complementary Medical Research*; 3: 1, 37–45.

Altman, D. (1994) The scandal of poor medical research. *British Medical Journal;* 308: 6924, 283–284.

Anthony, H. (1987) Some methodological problems in the assessment of complementary therapies. *Statistics in Medicine*; 6: 7, 761–771.

Ashkenazi, R. (1993) Multidimensional reflexology. *International Journal of Alternative and Complementary Medicine*; 11: 6, 8–12.

Barron, H. (1990) Towards better health with reflexology. *Nursing Standard*; 4: 40, 32–33.

Beckwith, C. (1993) The concept of touch as an aspect of therapeutic nursing. *Complementary Therapies in Medicine*; 1: 4, 211–214.

Benoussan, A. (1991) *The Vital Meridian*. Edinburgh: Churchill Livingstone.

Bettelheim, B. (1986) *The Informed Heart*. London: Penguin.

Betts, T. (1996) The fragrant breeze: the role of aromatherapy in treating epilepsy. *Aromatherapy Quarterly*; 51: 25–27.

Birch, S. (1997) Issues to consider in determining an adequate treatment in a clinical trial of acupuncture. *Complementary Therapies in Medicine*; 5: 8–12.

Birch, S. (1998) Diversity and acupuncture: acupuncture is not a coherent or historically stable tradition. In: Vickers, A. (ed) *Examining Complementary Medicine*. Cheltenham: Stanley Thornes.

Bosiger, C. (1989) Vacuflex reflexology shows the system is successful in clearing back pain. *Journal of Alternative and Complementary Medicine*; 7: 8, 25–26.

Botting, D. (1997) Review of literature on the effectiveness of reflexology. *Complementary Therapies in Nursing and Midwifery*; 3: 5, 123–130.

Buchbauer, G. (1992) *Biological Effects of Fragrances and Essential Oils* (paper from the 12th International Congress of Flavours, Fragrances and Essential Oils in Vienna, Austria). London: British Library.

Buchbauer, G., Jirovetz, L., Jager, W. (1991) Aromatherapy: evidence for sedative effects of the essential oil of lavender after inhalation. *Zeitschrift der Naturforschung*; 4 (c): 1067–1072.

Buchbauer, G., Jirovetz, L., Jager, W. (1992) Passiflora and lime blossoms: motility effects after inhalation of the essential oils and of some of the main constituents in animal experiment. *Archive of Pharmacology*; 325: 247–248.

Buchbauer, G., Jirovetz, L., Jager, W. et al (1993) Fragrance compounds and essential oils with sedative effects upon inhalation. *Journal of Pharmaceutical Sciences*; 82: 6, 660–664.

Buckle, J. (1993) Aromatherapy: Does it matter which lavender oil is used? *Nursing Times*; 89: 20, 32–35.

Bulbrook, M. (1984) Bulbrook's model of therapeutic touch: one form of health and healing for the future. *The Canadian Nurse*; December: 30–34.

Castledine, G. (1997) Evidence-based nursing: where is the evidence? *British Journal of Nursing*; 6: 5, 290.

Clark, P., Clark, M. (1984) Therapeutic Touch: is there a scientific basis for the practice? *Nursing Research*; 33: 1, 37–41.

Coe, W., Ryken, K. (1979) Hypnosis and risk to human subjects. *American Psychologist*; 34: 8, 673–681.

Cox, C., Hayes, J. (1997) Reducing anxiety: the employment of Therapeutic Touch as a nursing intervention. *Complementary Therapies in Nursing and Midwifery*; 3: 6, 163–167.

Cox, C., Hayes, J. (1998) The experience of administering and receiving Therapeutic Touch in intensive care. *Complementary Therapies in Nursing and Midwifery*. 4: 5, 128–133.

Darley, M. (1995) Complementary therapies: the position of the UKCC. *Complementary Therapies in Nursing and Midwifery*; 1: 4, 106–109.

Eddy, D., Billings, J. (1992) The quality of medical evidence and medical practice. Paper prepared for the National Leadership Commission on Health Care. Cited in: Buckman, R., Sabbagh, K. (1993) *Magic or Medicine? An Investigation into Healing*. London: Macmillan.

Ernst, E. (1998) Single-case studies in complementary/alternative medicine research. *Complementary Therapies in Medicine*; 6: 2, 75–78.

Ernst, E., Barnes, J.U. (1998) Methodological approaches to investigate the safety of complementary medicine. *Complementary Therapies in Medicine*; 6: 115–121.

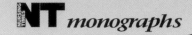

Evans, M. (1991) On the efficacy of anthroposophical medicines. *Complementary Medical Research*; 5: 2, 71–78.

Ewer, T., Stewart, D. (1986) Improvement in bronchial hyper-responsiveness in patients with moderate asthma after treatment with a hypnotic technique. A randomised controlled trial. *British Medical Journal*; 293: 1129–1132.

Fedoruk, R. (1985) Transfer of the relaxation response: Therapeutic Touch as a method for reduction of stress in premature neonates. *Dissertation Abstracts International*; 46: 978.

Field, T., Schanberg, S., Scarfidi, F. (1986) Tactile/kinesthetic stimulation effects on preterm neonates. *Pediatrics*; 77: 5, 654–658.

Fraser, J., Kerr, J. (1993) Physiological effects of back massage on elderly institutionalised patients. *Journal of Advanced Nursing*; 18: 2, 238–245.

Fowler, P., Wall, M. (1997) COSHH and CHIPS: ensuring the safety of aromatherapy. *Complementary Therapies in Medicine*; 5: 2, 112–115.

Fowler, P. Wall, M. (1998) Aromatherapy: control of substances hazardous to health (COSHH) and assessment of the chemical risk. *Complementary Therapies in Medicine*; 6: 2, 86–93.

Fulder, S. (1997) *The Handbook of Alternative and Complementary Medicine: The Essential Health Companion*. London: Vermillion.

Green, C. (1996) A reflection of a Therapeutic Touch experience: case study 1. *Complementary Therapies in Nursing and Midwifery*; 2: 5, 122–125.

Goodwin, H. (1992) Reflex zone therapy. In: Rankin-Box, D. (ed) *Complementary Health Therapies: A Guide for Nurses and the Caring Professions*. London: Chapman and Hall.

Grayson, L. (1997) *Evidence-Based Medicine*. London: The British Library.

Griffiths, P. (1995) Vacu-reflexology. In: Rankin-Box, D. (ed) *The Nurse's Handbook of Complementary Therapies*. Edinburgh: Churchill Livingstone.

Hammerschlag, R., Morris, M. (1997) Clinical trials comparing acupuncture with biomedical standard care: a criteria-based evaluation of research design and reporting. *Complementary Therapies in Medicine*; 5: 3, 133–140.

Hardy, M. (1991) Sweet-scented dreams. *International Journal of Aromatherapy*; 3: 1, 12–13.

Harrison, L., Leeper, J., Yoon, M. (1990) Effects of early parent touch on preterm infants' heart rates and arterial oxygen saturation levels. *Journal of Advanced Nursing*; 15: 8, 877–885.

Heron, J. (1986) Critique of conventional research methodology. *Complementary Medical Research*; 1: 12–22.

Heidt, P. (1981) Effects of Therapeutic Touch on anxiety levels of hospitalised patients. *Nursing Research*; 30: 1, 32–37.

Hesse, J., Mogelvang, B., Simonsen, H. (1994) Acupuncture versus metoprolol in migraine prophylactics: a randomised trial of trigger point inactivation. *Journal of Internal Medicine*; 235: 5, 451–456.

Ingham, E. (1984) *Stories Feet Have Told*. St Petersburg, Florida: Ingham Publishing Corporation.

Jager, W., Buchbauer, G., Jirovetz, L., et al (1992) Evidence of the sedative effect of neroli oil, citronella and phenylethyl acetate on mice. *Journal of Essential Oil Research*; 4: 387–394.

Keller, E., Bzdek, U. (1986) Effects of Therapeutic Touch on tension headache pain. *Nursing Research*; 2: 35, 101–105.

Kleijnen, J., Ter Riet, G., Knipschild, P. (1991) Acupuncture and asthma: a review of controlled trials. *Thorax*; 46: 11, 799–802.

Knape, J. (1998) Complementary therapies and the registered nurse, midwife and health visitor. *Complementary Therapies in Nursing and Midwifery*; 4: 2, 54–56.

Kohen, D., Colwell, S., Heimel, A., Olness, K. (1984) The use of relaxation/mental imagery in the management of 505 pediatric behavioural encounters. *Journal of Developmental and Behavioural Pediatrics*; 5: 1, 21–25.

Kramer, N. (1990) Comparison of Therapeutic Touch and casual touch in stress reduction of hospitalised children. *Pediatric Nursing*; 16: 5, 483–485.

Krieger, D. (1974) Healing by the laying on of hands as a facilitator of bioenergetic change: the response of *in vivo* human haemoglobin. *Psychoenergetic Systems*; 1: 121–129.

Lafuente, A., Noquera, M., Puye, C. et al (1990) Effekt der Reflexonenbehandlung am Fuß bezüglich der prophylaktischen Behandlung mit Flunarizin bei an Cephalea-Kopfschmerzen leidenden Patienten. *Erfahrungsheilkunde*; 39: 11, 713–715.

Leibrich, J. (1990) Measurement of efficacy: a case for holistic research. *Complementary Medical Research*; 4: 1, 21–25.

Levine, E. (1980) Indirect suggestions through personalised fairy tales for the treatment of childhood insomnia. *American Journal of Clinical Hypnosis*; 23: 1, 57–63.

Lewith, G. (1997) The use and abuse of evidence-based medicine: an example from general practice. In: Ernst, E. (ed) *Complementary Medicine: An Objective Appraisal*. Oxford: Butterworth-Heinemann.

Lewith, G. (1998) Misconceptions about research in complementary medicine. In: Vickers, A. (ed) *Examining Complementary Medicine*. Cheltenham, Glos: Stanley Thornes.

Lewith, G. (1984) How effective is acupuncture in the management of pain? *Journal of the Royal College of General Practitioners*; 34: 262, 275–278.

Lewith, G. (1995) The treatment of tobacco addiction. *Complementary Therapies in Medicine*; 3: 3, 142–145.

Notes

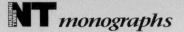

Notes

Lewith, G., Kenyon, J. (1984) Physiological and psychological explanations for the mechanism of acupuncture as a treatment for chronic pain. *Social Science and Medicine*; 19: 12, 1367–1378.

Lis-Balchin, M., Hart, S., Deans, S. (1996) Comparison of the pharmacological and antimicrobial action of commercial plant essential oils. *Journal of Herbs, Spices and Medicinal Plants*; 4: 2, 69–86.

Lis-Balchin, M. (1997) Essential oils and aromatherapy: their role in modern healing. *Journal of the Royal Society of Health*; 117: 5, 324–329.

Mantle, F. (1996) Safe practices. *Nursing Times*; 92: 6, 36–38.

Mantle, F. (1997) Implementing evidence in practice. *British Journal of Community Health Nursing*; 2: 1, 36–39.

McGourty, H. (1993) *How to Evaluate Complementary Therapies: A Literature Review*. Liverpool: Public Health Observatory.

Meehan, T. (1993) Therapeutic Touch and postoperative pain: A Rogerian research study. *Nursing Science Quarterly*; 6: 2, 69–78.

Morrison, J. (1988) Chronic asthma and improvement with relaxation induced by hypnotherapy. *Journal of the Royal Society of Medicine*; 81: 12, 701–704.

Motha, G., McGrath, J. (1994) *The Effects of Reflexology on Labour Outcome. International Association of Reflexologists Reflexology Research Reports*. London: Association of Reflexologists.

Muir Gray, J. (1997) *Evidence-Based Health Care How to Make Policy and Management Decisions*. Edinburgh: Churchill Livingstone.

NHS Executive (1996) *Promoting Clinical Effectiveness: A Framework for Action*. Leeds: NHSE.

Oehler, J. (1985) Examining the issue of tactile stimulation for preterm infants. *Neonatal Network*; 4: 3, 25–33.

Oleson, T., Flocco, W. (1993) Randomised controlled study of premenstrual symptoms treated with ear, hand and foot reflexology. *Obstetrics and Gynaecology*; 28: 6, 906–911.

Olness, K. (1975) The use of self-hypnosis in the treatment of childhood nocturnal enuresis. A report on 40 patients. *Clinical Pediatrics*; 14: 3, 273–279.

Olness, K., Gardner, G. (1978) Some guidelines for the use of hypnotherapy in pediatrics. *Pediatrics*; 62: 2, 228–233.

Parkes, B. (1985) *Therapeutic Touch as an Intervention to Reduce Anxiety in Elderly Hospitalised Patients (doctoral dissertation)*. Austin, Texas: University of Texas.

Porter, J. (1975) Guided fantasy as a treatment for childhood insomnia. *Australian and New Zealand Journal of Psychiatry*; 9: 3, 169–172.

Powell, L. (1974) The effect of extra stimulation and maternal involvement on the development of low-birthweight infants and on maternal behaviour. *Child Development*; 45: 1, 106–113.

Quinn, J. (1982) An investigation into the effect of Therapeutic Touch done without physical contact on state anxiety of hospital cardiovascular patients. *Dissertation Abstracts International*; 43: 17976.

Quinn, J. (1989) Therapeutic Touch as energy exchange: replication and extension. *Nursing Science Quarterly*; 2: 2, 79–87.

Rampes, H., James, R. (1995) Complications of acupuncture. *Acupuncture in Medicine*; 13: 1, 26–33.

Rampes, H., Mortimer, A. (1997) Letter to the editor. *Complementary Therapies in Medicine*; 13: 1, 26–3.

Rankin-Box, D. (1995) *The Nurse's Handbook of Complementary Therapies*. Edinburgh: Churchill Livingstone.

Resch, K., Ernst, E. (1997) Research methodologies in complementary medicine: making sure it works. In: Ernst, E. (ed) *Complementary Therapies and Objective Appraisal*. Oxford: Butterworth-Heinemann.

RCN (1996) *Clinical Effectiveness*. London: RCN.

Sackett, D., Rosenberg, W., Muir Gray, J. et al (1996) Evidence-based medicine: what it is and what it isn't. *British Medical Journal*; 312: 7023, 71–72.

Scarfeldi, F., Field, T. et al (1993) Factors which predict which preterm infants benefit from massage therapy. *Journal of Developmental and Behavioural Paediatrics*. 14: 3, 3–8.

Scoville, W.B., Milner, B. (1957) Loss of recent memory after hippocampal lesions. *Journal of Neurology, Neurosurgery and Psychiatry*; 20: 11–21.

Silagy, C., Mant, D., Fowler, G. et al (1994) Meta-analysis of efficacy of nicotine replacement therapy in smoking cessation. *Lancet*; 343: 8890, 139–142.

Spoerke, D. (1989) Toxicity of homoeopathic products. *Veterinary and Human Toxicology*; 31: 3, 259–260.

Schwartz, J. (1988) Evaluation of acupuncture as a treatment for smoking. *American Journal of Acupuncture*; 16: 135–142.

Staebler, F., Wheeler, J., Young, J. et al (1994) Why research into acupuncture has proved difficult. Strategies for the Council for Acupuncture UK to overcome the problem. *Complementary Therapies in Medicine*; 2: 2, 86–92.

Stevensen, C. (1994) The psychophysiological effects of aromatherapy masssage following cardiac surgery. *Complementary Therapies in Medicine*; 2: 1, 27–35.

Swayne, J. (1998) Homeopathic therapeutics: many dimensions or meaningless diversity? In: Vickers, A. (ed) *Examining Complementary Medicine*. Cheltenham, Glos.: Stanley Thornes.

Ter Riet, G., Kleijnen, J., Knipschild, P. (1990a) Acupuncture and chronic pain: a criteria-based meta-analysis. *Journal of Clinical Epidemiology*; 43: 11, 1191–1199.

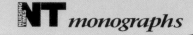

Ter Riet, G., Kleijnen, J., Knipschild, P. (1990b) Meta-analysis of studies into the effect of acupuncture on addiction. *British Journal of General Practice;* 40: 338, 379–382.

Thayer, M. (1990) Touching with intent: using Therapeutic Touch. *Pediatric Nursing;* 16: 1, 70–72.

Thomas, M. (1989) Fancy footwork. *Nursing Times;* 85: 41, 42–44.

Tilton, P. (1980) Hypnotic treatment of a child with thumb-sucking, enuresis and encopresis. *American Journal of Clinical Hypnosis;* 22: 4, 238–340.

Trevelyan, J., Booth, B. (1994) *Complementary Medicine for Nurses, Midwives and Health Visitors.* London: Macmillan.

UKCC (1992) *Standards for the Administration of Medicines Section 39.* London: UKCC.

Vickers, A. (1996) *Massage and Aromatherapy: A Guide for Health Professionals.* London: Chapman and Hall.

Vickers, A. (1997) Research paradigms in mainstream and complementary medicine. In: Ernst, E. (ed) *Complementary Medicine: An Objective Appraisal.* Oxford: Butterworth-Heinemann.

Vincent, C., Richardson, P. (1987) Acupuncture for some common disorders: a review of evaluative research. *Journal of the Royal College of General Practitioners;* 37: 77–81.

Wirth, D. (1995) Complementary healing intervention and dermal wound re-epithelisation: an overview. *International Journal of Psychosomatics;* 42: 1–4, 48–53.

Further reading

Dossey, L. (1995) How should complementary therapies be evaluated? An examination of fundamentals. *Alternative Therapies in Health and Medicine;* I: 2, 6–10/79–85.

Ernst, E. (ed) (1996) *Complementary Medicine: An Objective Appraisal.* Oxford: Butterworth Heinemann.

Fulder, S. (1996) *The Handbook of Alternative and Complementary Medicine.* London: Vermillion Press.

Mercer, G., Long, A., Smith, I. (1995) *Researching and Evaluating Complementary Therapies: The State of the Debate.* Leeds: Nuffield Institute for Health, University of Leeds.

Micozzi, M. (1996) *Fundamentals of Complementary and Alternative Medicine.* Edinburgh: Churchill Livingstone.

NHS Centre for Reviews and Dissemination (1996) *Undertaking Systematic Reviews of Research on Effectiveness.* York: University of York.

Rankin-Box, D. (1993) Innovations in practice: complementary therapies in nursing. *Complementary Therapies in Medicine;* 1: 1, 30–33.

Rees, R. (1995) CISCOM, the Centralised Information Service for Complementary Medicine. *Complementary Therapies in Medicine;* 3: 3, 183–186.

Research Council for Complementary Medicine (1995) *Searching for Published Information in Complementary Therapies: A Resource Guide.* London: RCCM.

Tiran, D., Mack, S. (1999) *Complementary Therapies for Pregnancy and Childbirth.* London: Baillière Tindall.

Vickers, A. (1998) *Examining Complementary Medicine.* Cheltenham: Stanley Thornes.

Vickers, A., Rees, R. (1995) Literature searching in complementary medicine research. *Complementary Therapies in Nursing and Midwifery;* 1: 6, 175–177.

Vincent, C., Furnham, A. (1997) *Complementary Medicine: A Research Perspective.* Chichester: Wiley and Sons.

Vincent, C., Furnham, A. (1997) The perceived efficacy of complementary and orthodox medicine: a replication. *Complementary Therapies in Medicine;* 5: 2, 85–89.

Aromatherapy

Cawthorn, A. (1995) A review of the literature surrounding the research into aromatherapy. *Complementary Therapies in Nursing and Midwifery;* 1: 4, 118–120.

Corner, J., Cawley, I., Hildebrand, S. (1995) An evaluation of the use of massage and essential oils on the well-being of cancer patients. *International Journal of Palliative Nursing;* 1: 2, 67–73.

Davis, P. (1996) *Aromatherapy: An A-Z.* Saffron Walden, Essex: C.W. Daniels.

Evans, B. (1995) An audit into the effects of aromatherapy massage and the cancer patient in palliative and terminal care. *Complementary Therapies in Medicine;* 3: 4, 239–241.

Lis-Balchin, M. (1995) *Aroma Science: The Chemistry and Bioactivity of Essential Oils.* East Horsley, Sussex: Amberwood Publishing.

Price, S., Price, L. (1995) *Aromatherapy for Health Professionals.* Edinburgh: Churchill Livingstone.

Ruckle, J. (1997) *Clinical Aromatherapy.* London: Arnold.

Tiran, D. (1996) *Aromatherapy in Midwifery Practice.* London: Baillière Tindall.

Tisserand, R. (1994) *The Art of Aromatherapy.* Saffron Walden, Essex: C.W. Daniels.

Tisserand, R., Balacs, T. (1995) *Essential Oil Safety: A Guide for Health Care Professionals.* Edinburgh: Churchill Livingstone.

Notes

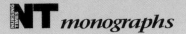
Notes

Vickers, A. (1996) *Massage and Aromatherapy: A Guide for Health Professionals.* London: Chapman and Hall.

Reflexology

Eriksen, L. (1995) Using reflexology to relieve chronic constipation. In: Danish Reflexologists Association. *A Collection of Articles.* Copenhagen, Denmark: Danish Reflexologists Association.

Griffiths, P. (1996) Reflexology. *Complementary Therapies in Nursing and Midwifery*; 2: 1, 13–16.

Wiran, D. (1996) The use of complementary therapies in midwifery: a focus on reflexology. *Complementary Therapies in Nursing and Midwifery*; 2: 2, 32–37.

Hypnosis

Gibson, H., Heap, M. (1991) *Hypnosis in Therapy.* London: Lawrence Erlbaum Associates.

Heap, M., Dryden, W. (1991) *Hypnotherapy: A Handbook.* Milton Keynes: Open University Press.

Olness, K., Kohen, D. (1996) *Hypnosis and Hypnotherapy with Children.* London: Guildford Press.

Acupuncture/traditional Chinese medicine

Gould, A. (1997) An introduction to the work of the acupuncture research resource centre and ARRCBASE: a bibliographic database of acupuncture practice and research. *Complementary Therapies in Medicine*; 57: 37, 168–171.

Joshi, Y. (1992) Acupuncture: a critical evaluation. *Journal of the Association of Physicians of India*; 49: 3, 184–189.

Kaptchuk, T. (1993) *Chinese Medicine: The Web that has no Weaver.* London: Rider.

McNamara, S., Xuan Ke, S. (1995) *Traditional Chinese Medicine. London*: Hamish Hamilton.

Sims, J. (1997) The mechanism for acupuncture analgesia: a review. *Complementary Therapies in Medicine*; 5: 2, 102–111.

Therapeutic Touch

Mills, A. (1996) Therapeutic Touch: case study of the application, documentation and outcome. *Complementary Therapies in Medicine*; 4: 2, 127–132.

Samarel, N. (1992) The experience of receiving Therapeutic Touch. *Journal of Advanced Nursing*; 17: 6, 651–657.

Sayre-Adams, J., Wright, S. (1996) *The Theory and Practice of Therapeutic Touch.* Edinburgh: Churchill Livingstone.

Wilson, D. (1995) Therapeutic Touch: foundations and current knowledge. *Alternative Health Practitioner*; 1: 1, 55–66.

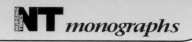

Notes

Notes

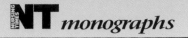

Notes

Notes